The Adventures of Baby Noah

By Samantha Pegues

Illustrated by Diana Design

Published by: Pegues Enterprises, LLC
ISBN: 9780692085585
www.samanthapegues.org

Dedication

This book is dedicated to Baby Jaxson LaTrell Egerson. Baby Jaxson passed away on November 29, 2017 due to heart complications. May his sweet smile always fill the void in the hearts of those who loved him.

Hi! My name is Baby Noah! I can’t wait to be born! My mom doesn’t know it, but I can feel and hear everything that goes on around her. Even the bad words!

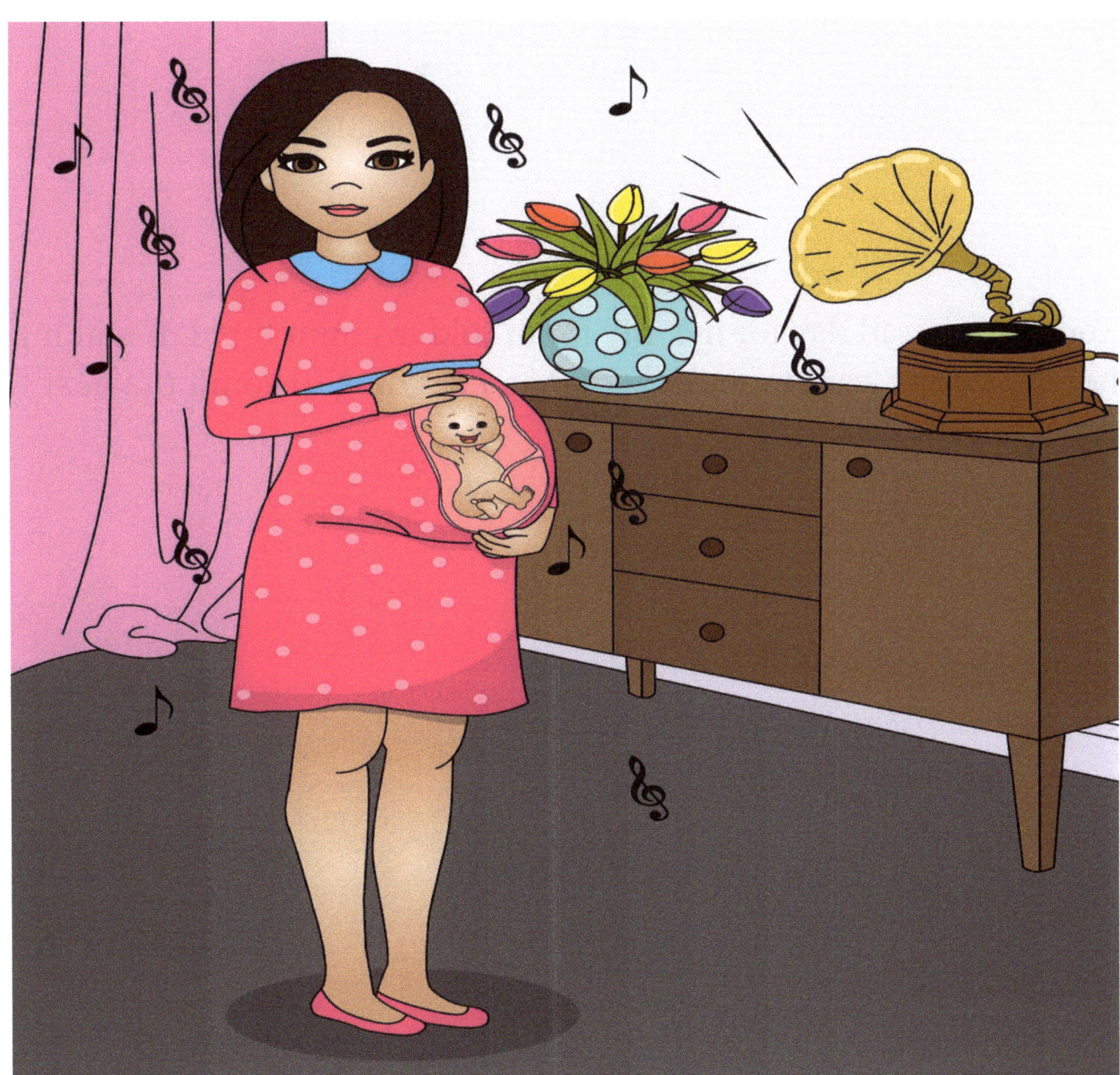

Today was a sad day for me. My mom told my aunt that I'm making her fat. I don't want to make her fat so I'm going to vomit the next time that she eats.

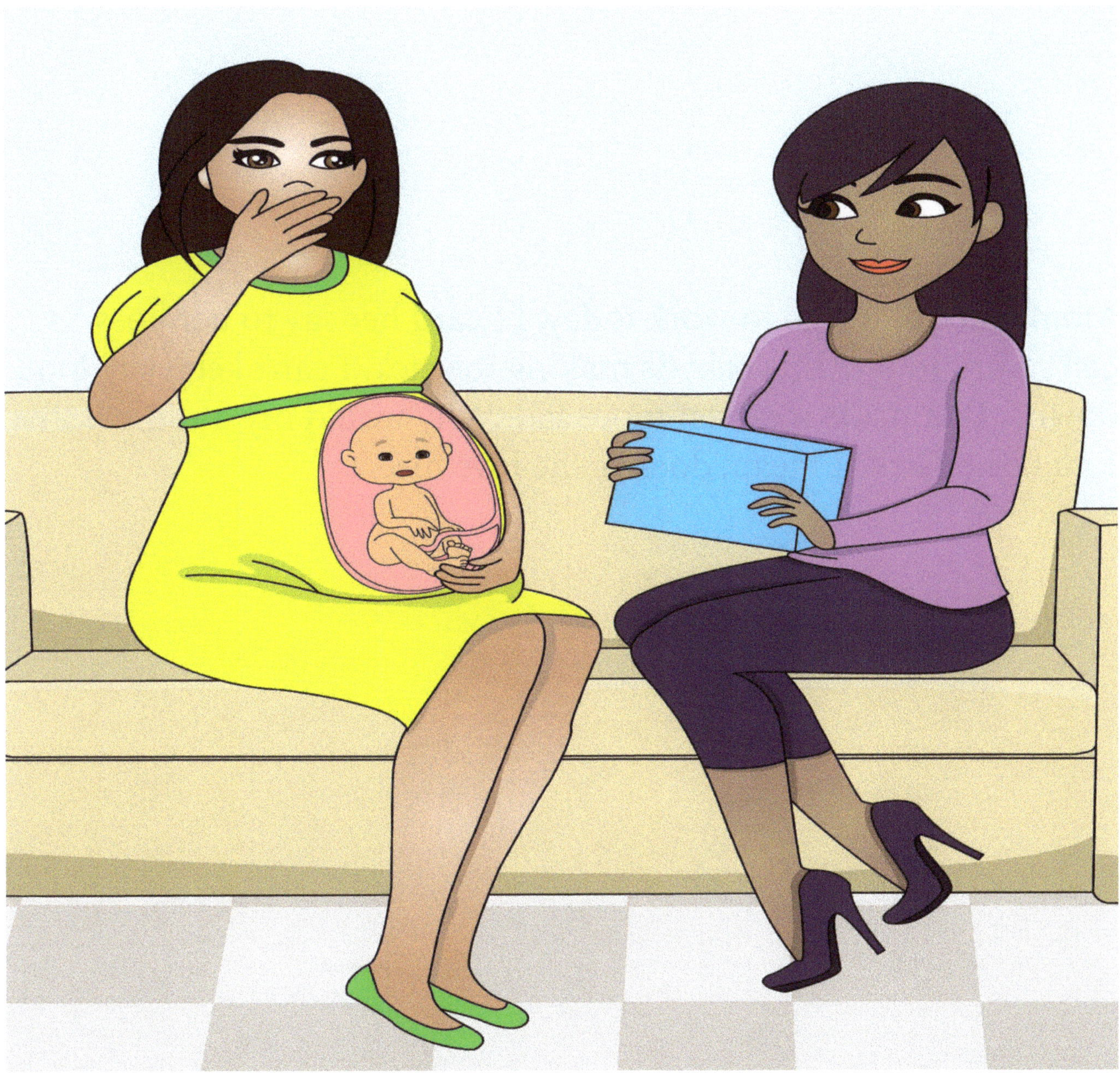

Mom and I didn't go to work today. I heard her say to her boss, "I can't work today. This baby is making me sick. I can't keep any food down." That made me even more sad. Why would my mom say that I make her sick? I mean, doesn't she love me?

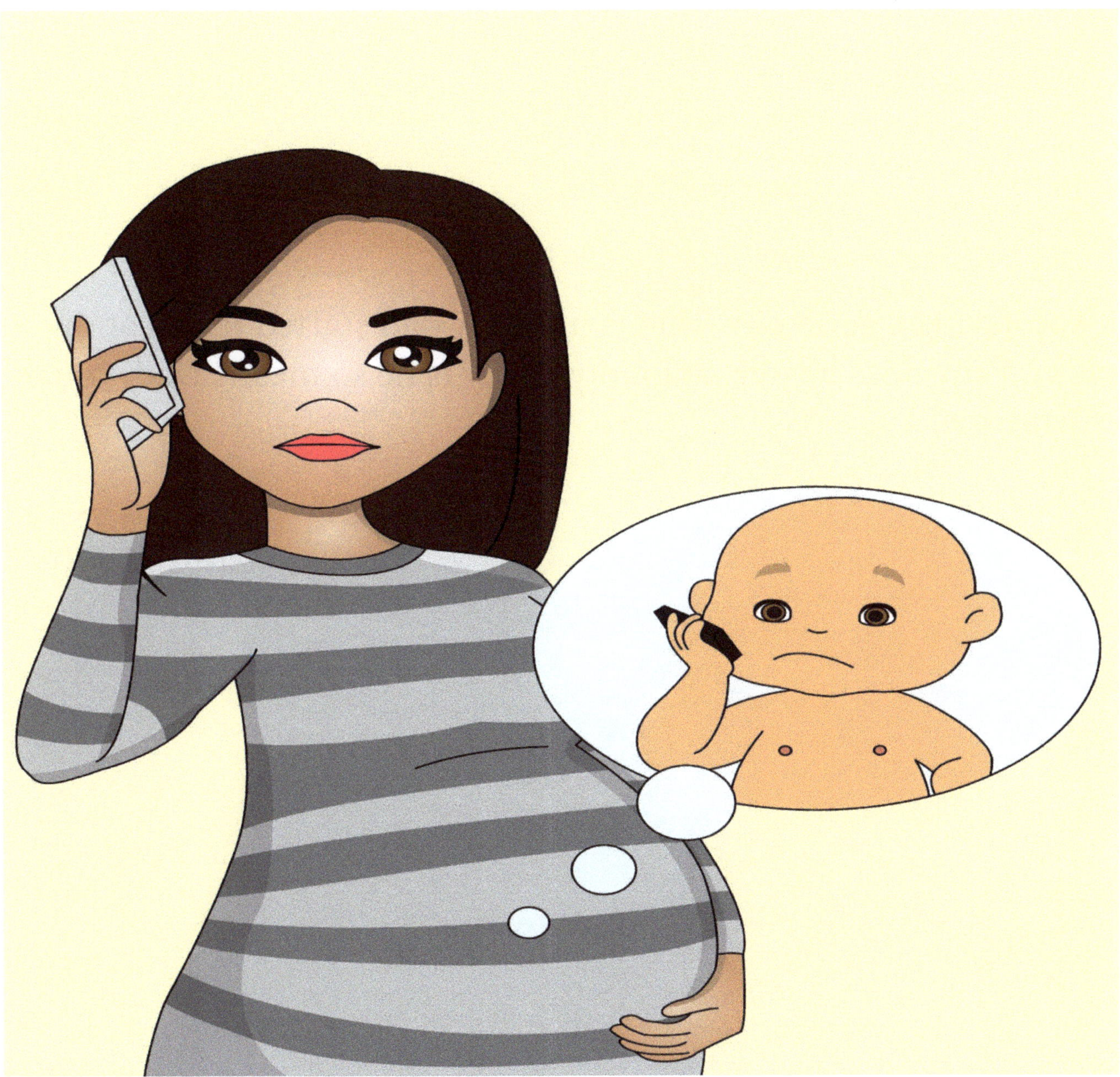

I was having a good day. That is until my dad started to yell at my mom. Why does he talk so loudly? Why is he so mean? Dad, you're scaring me!

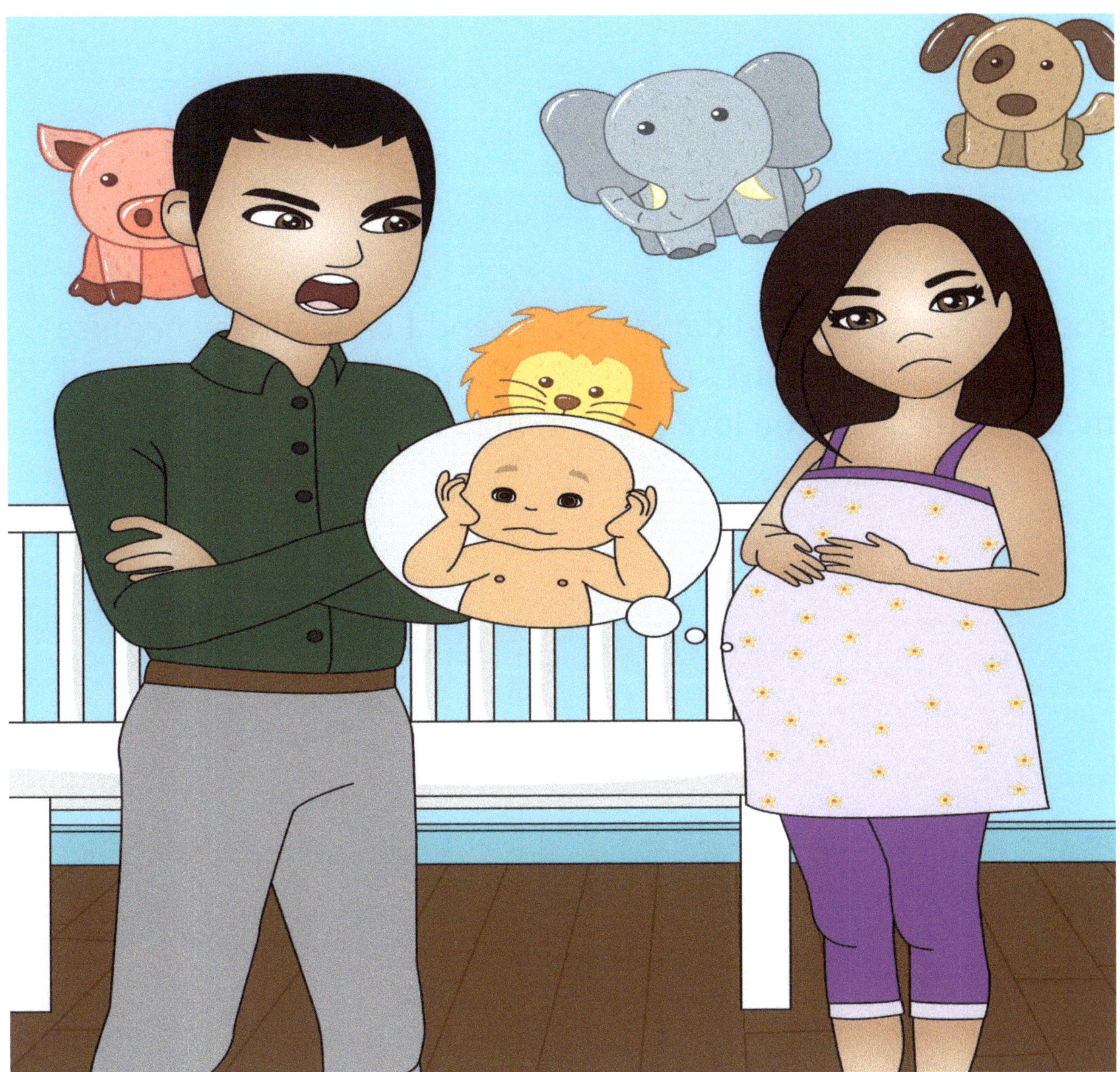

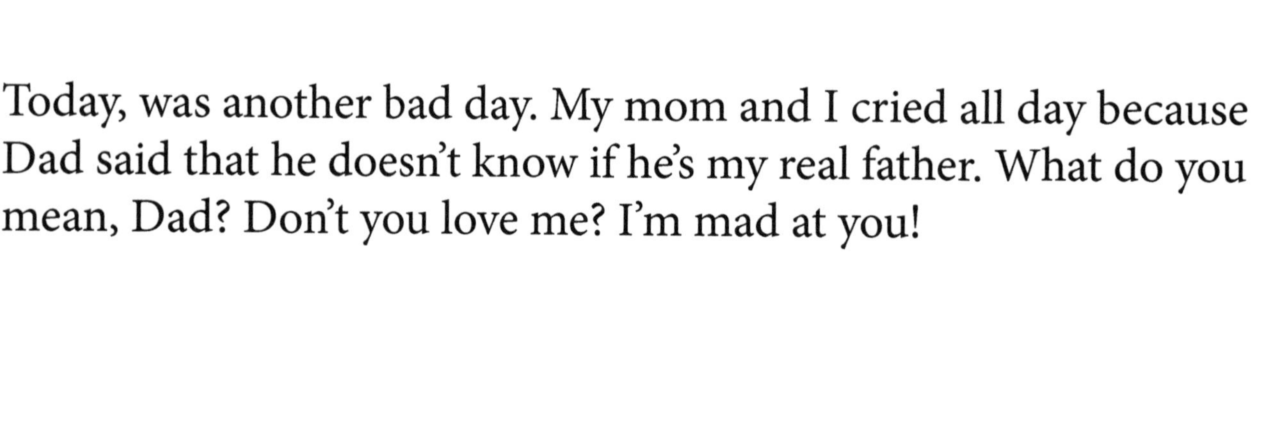

Today, was another bad day. My mom and I cried all day because Dad said that he doesn't know if he's my real father. What do you mean, Dad? Don't you love me? I'm mad at you!

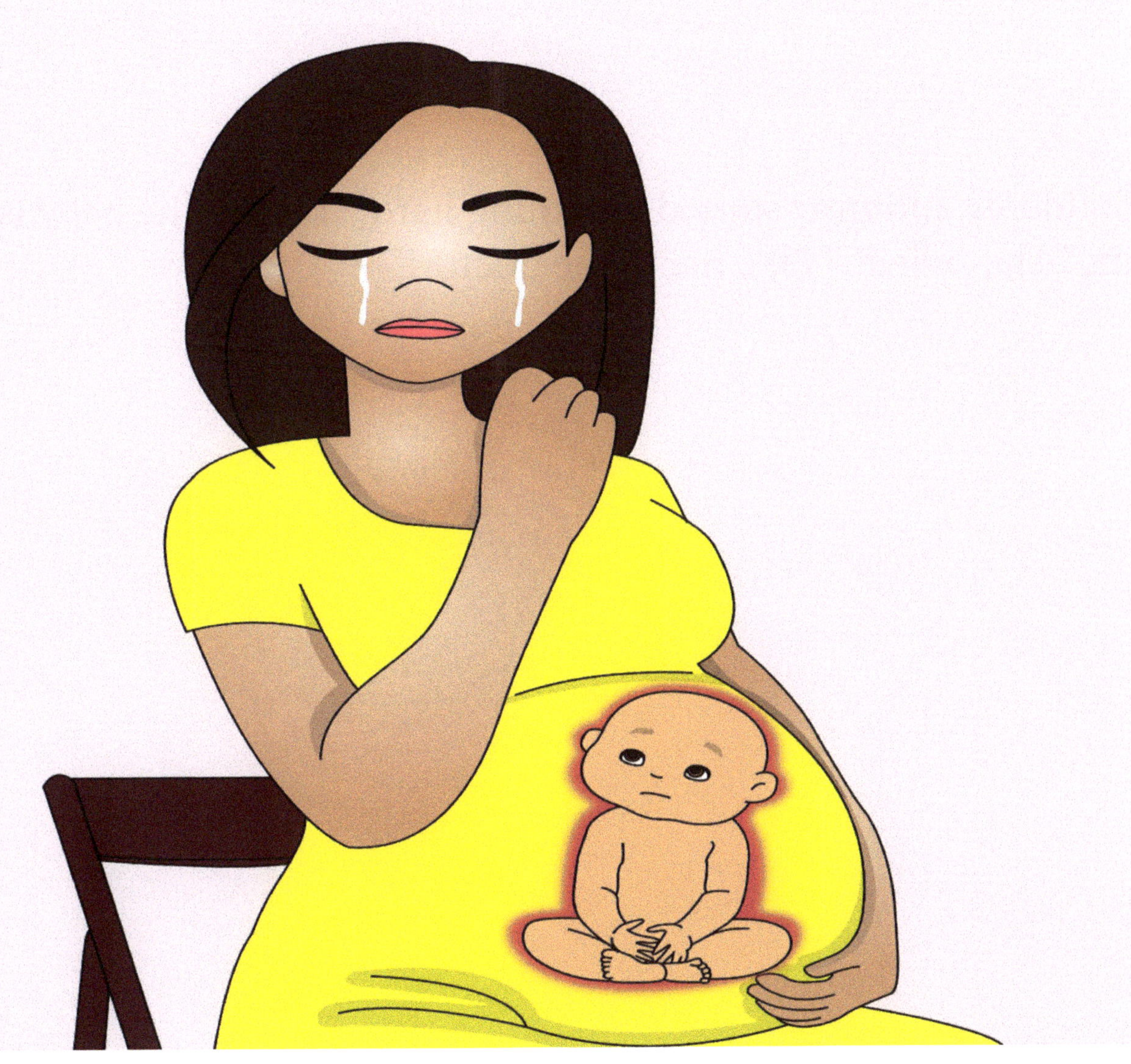

Suddenly, mommy started breathing hard. “I think the baby is com-ing,” she yelled! “Take me to the doctor!”

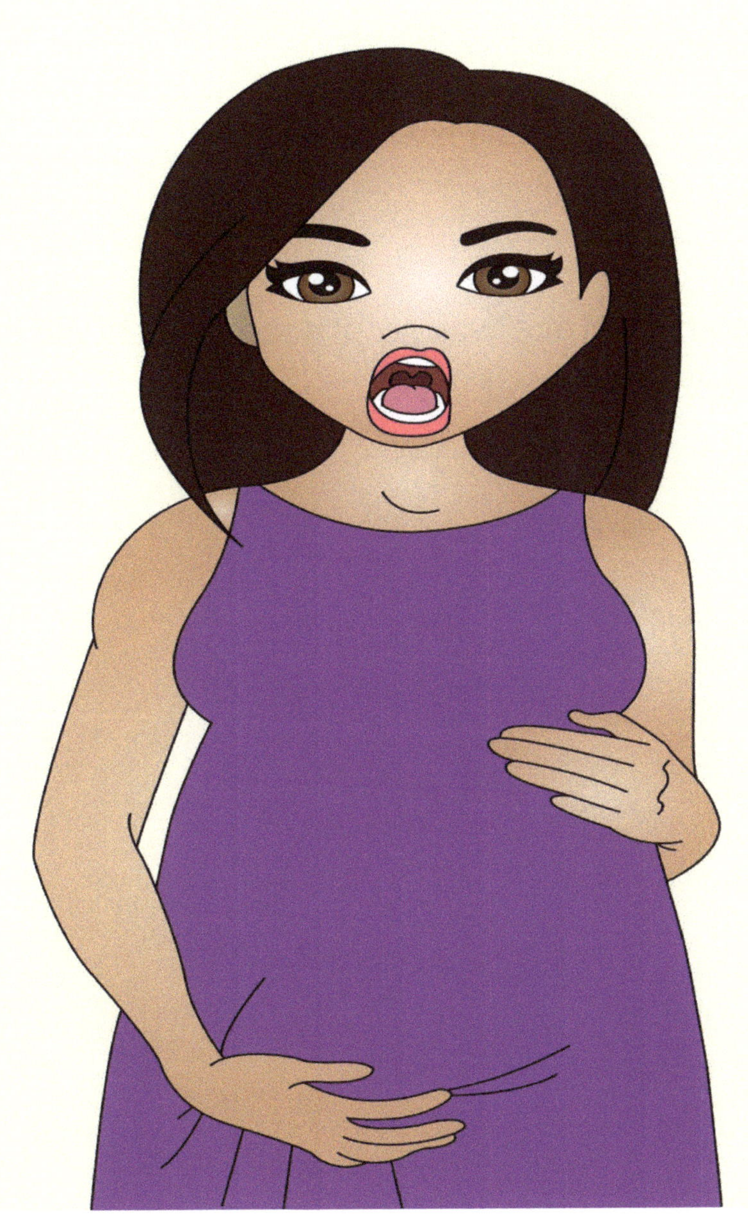

The ride in the ambulance was so much fun! The sirens were really loud and we were going so fast!

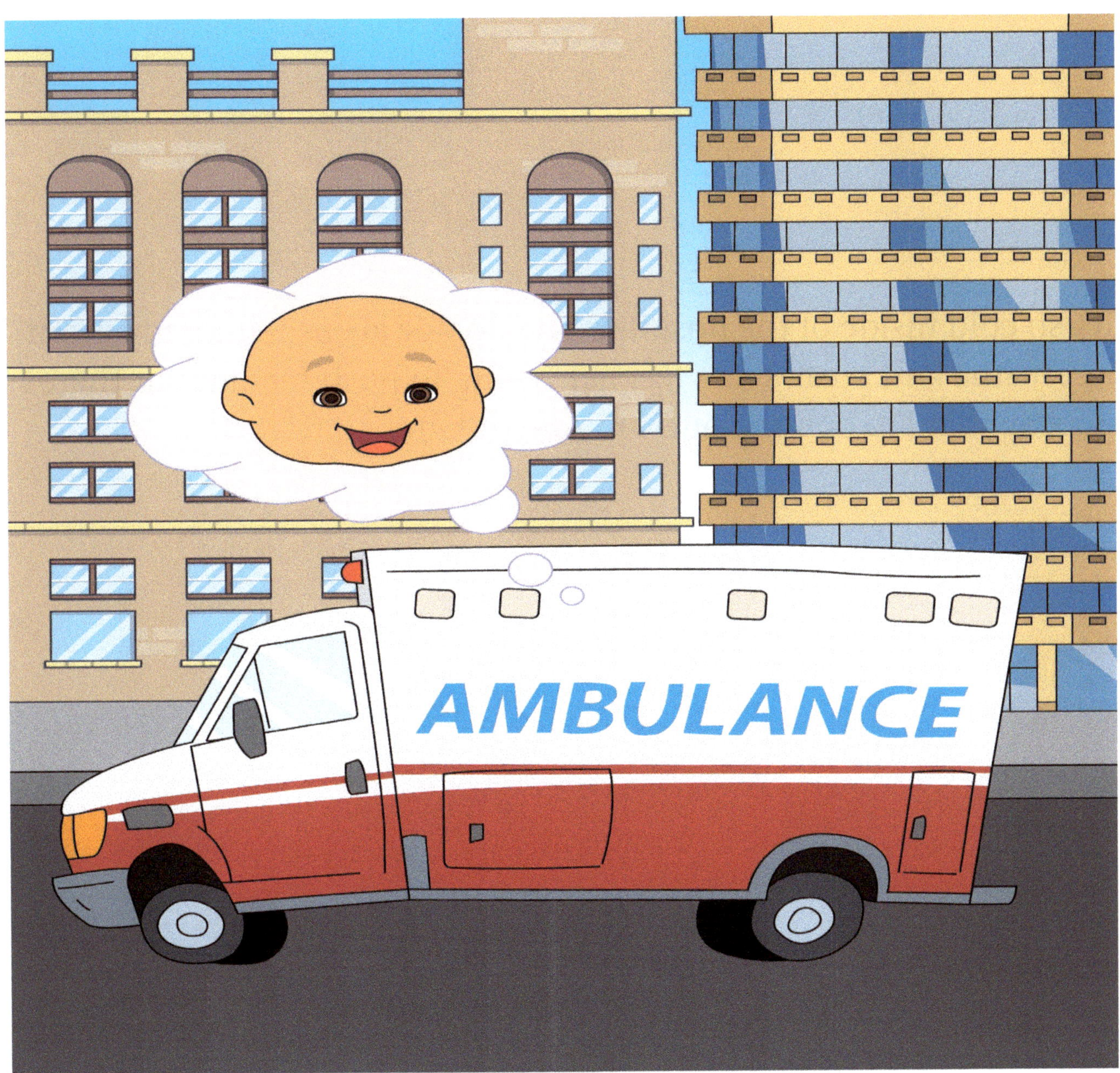
AMBULANCE

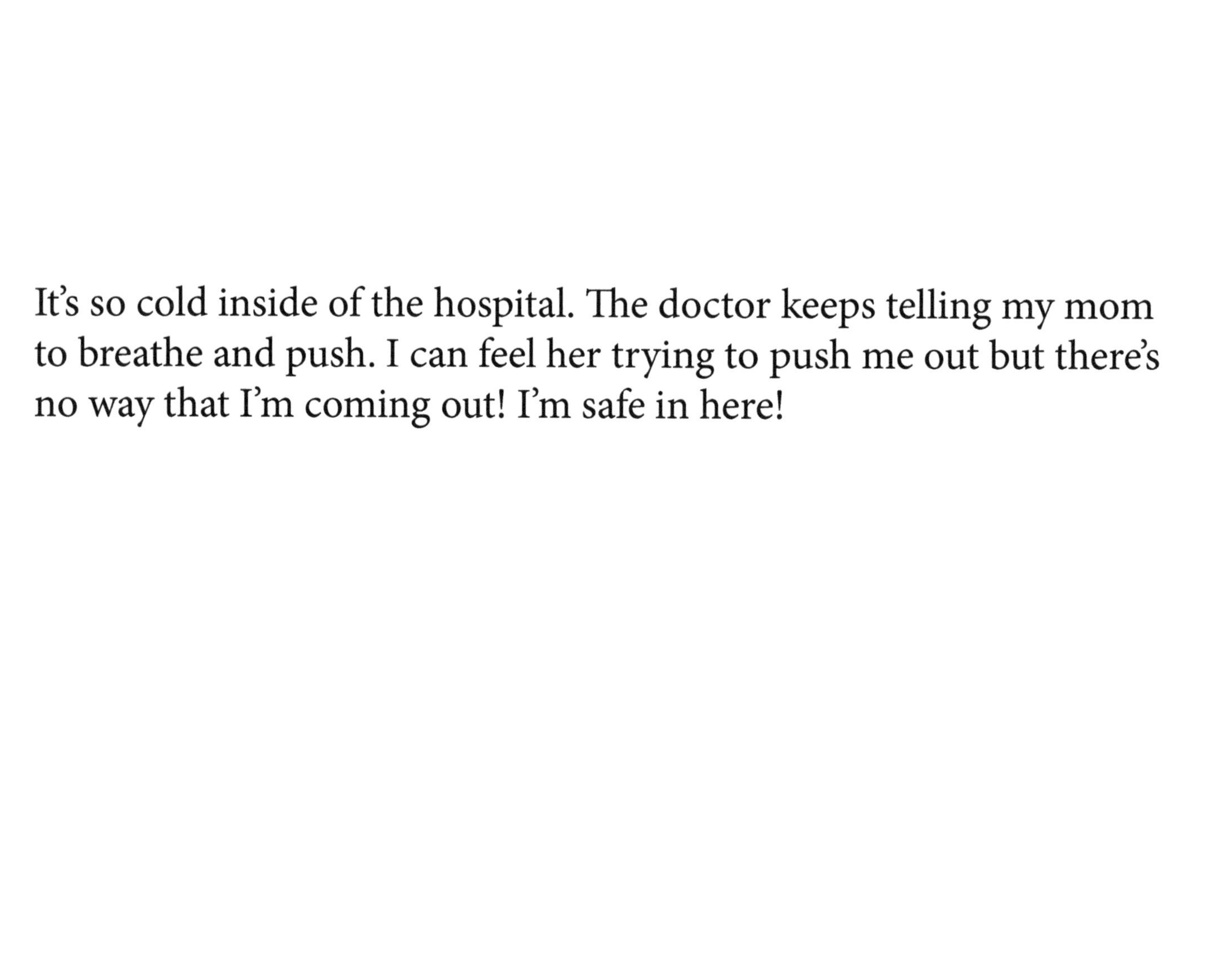

It’s so cold inside of the hospital. The doctor keeps telling my mom to breathe and push. I can feel her trying to push me out but there’s no way that I’m coming out! I’m safe in here!

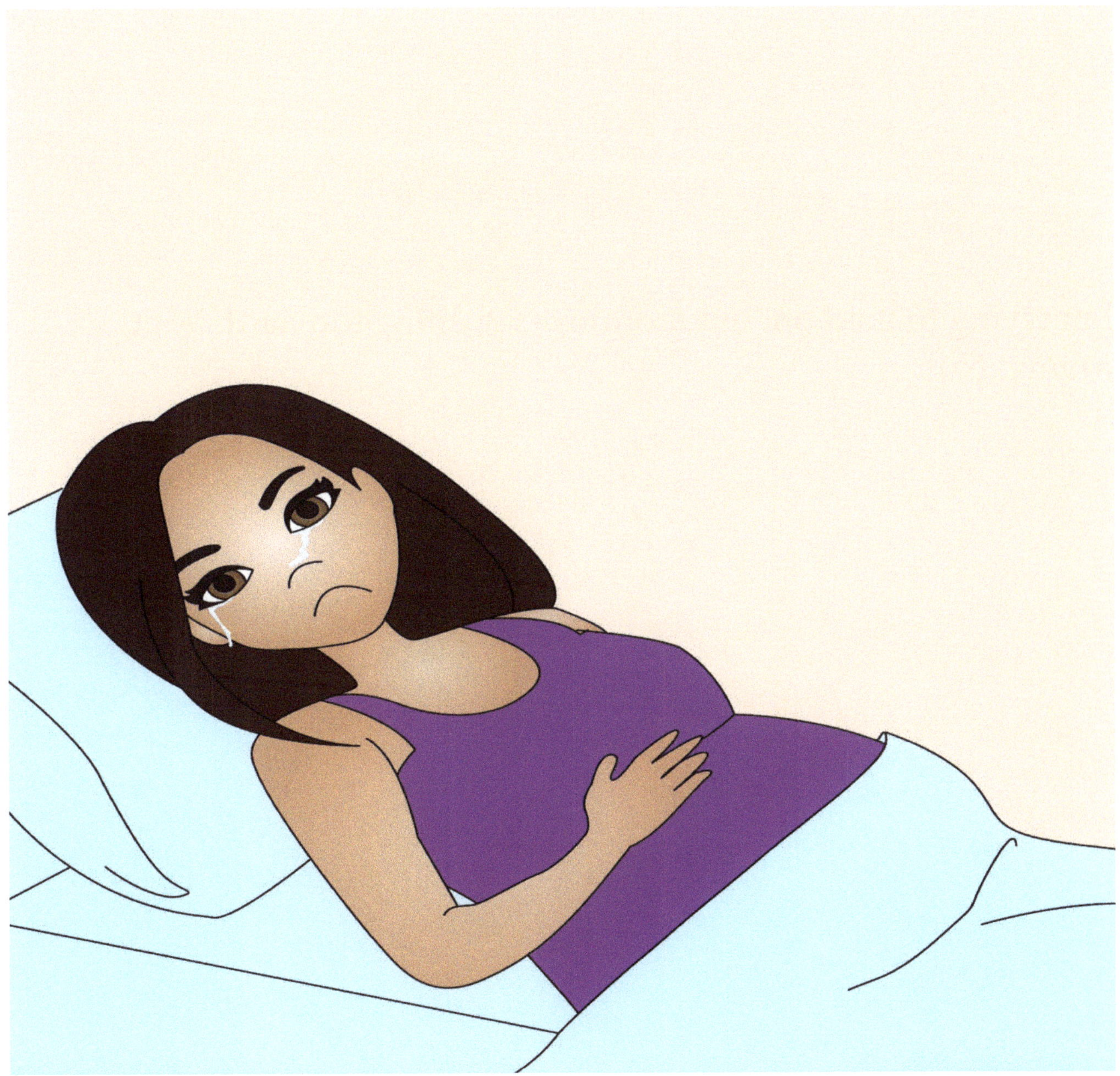

I'm trying to hold on, but mommy is pushing too hard. Wait, Mama! No!

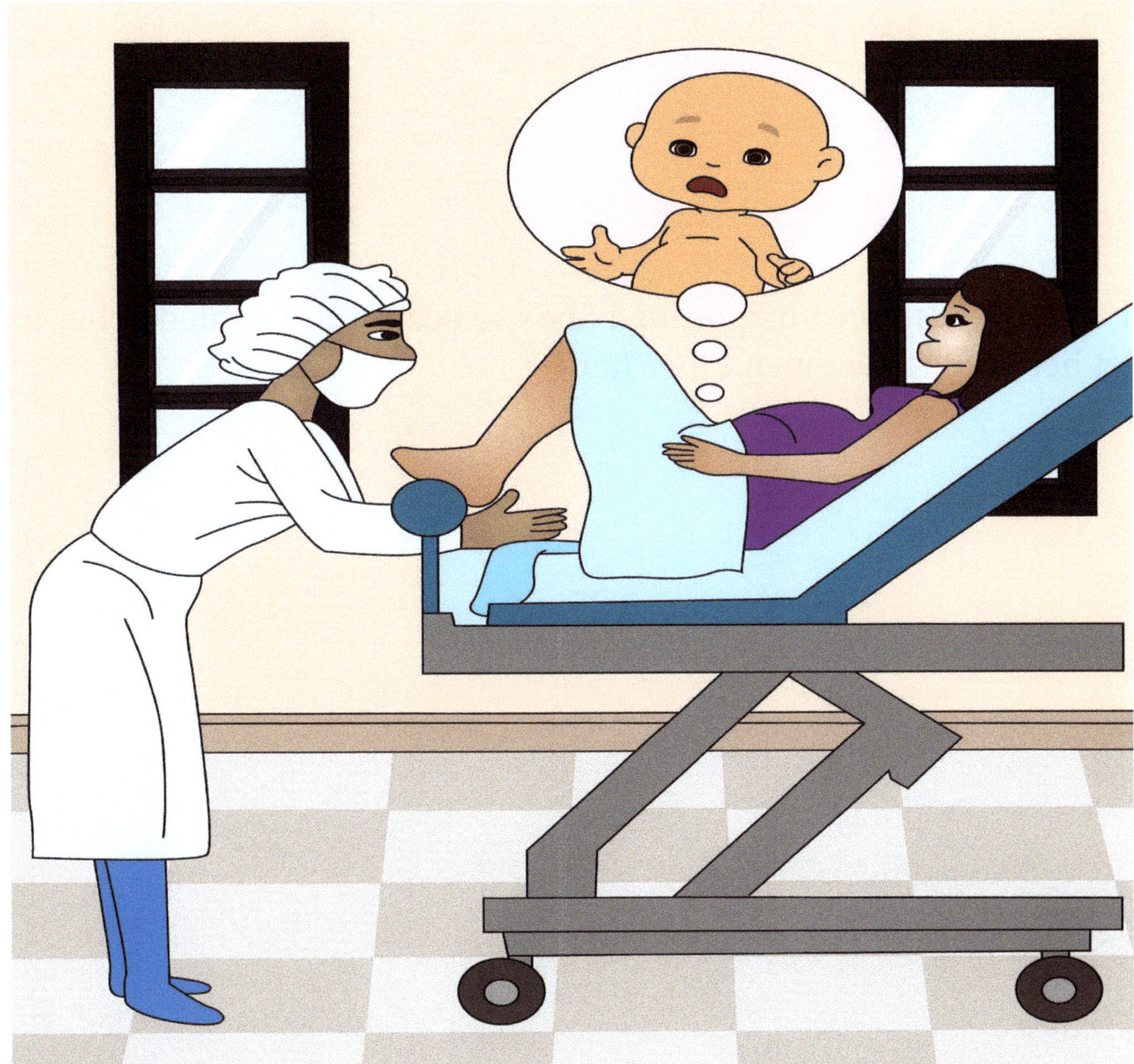

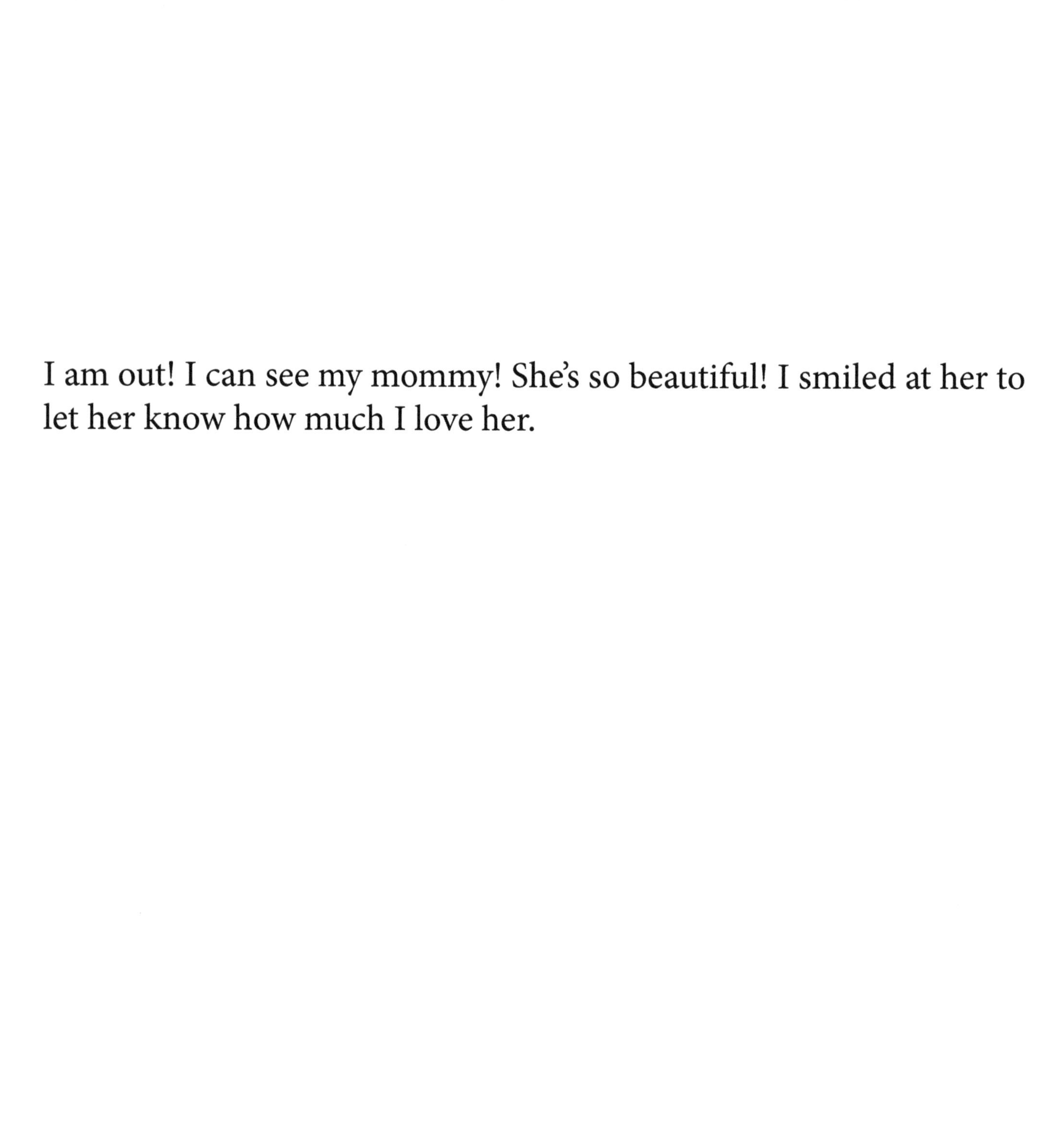

I am out! I can see my mommy! She's so beautiful! I smiled at her to let her know how much I love her.

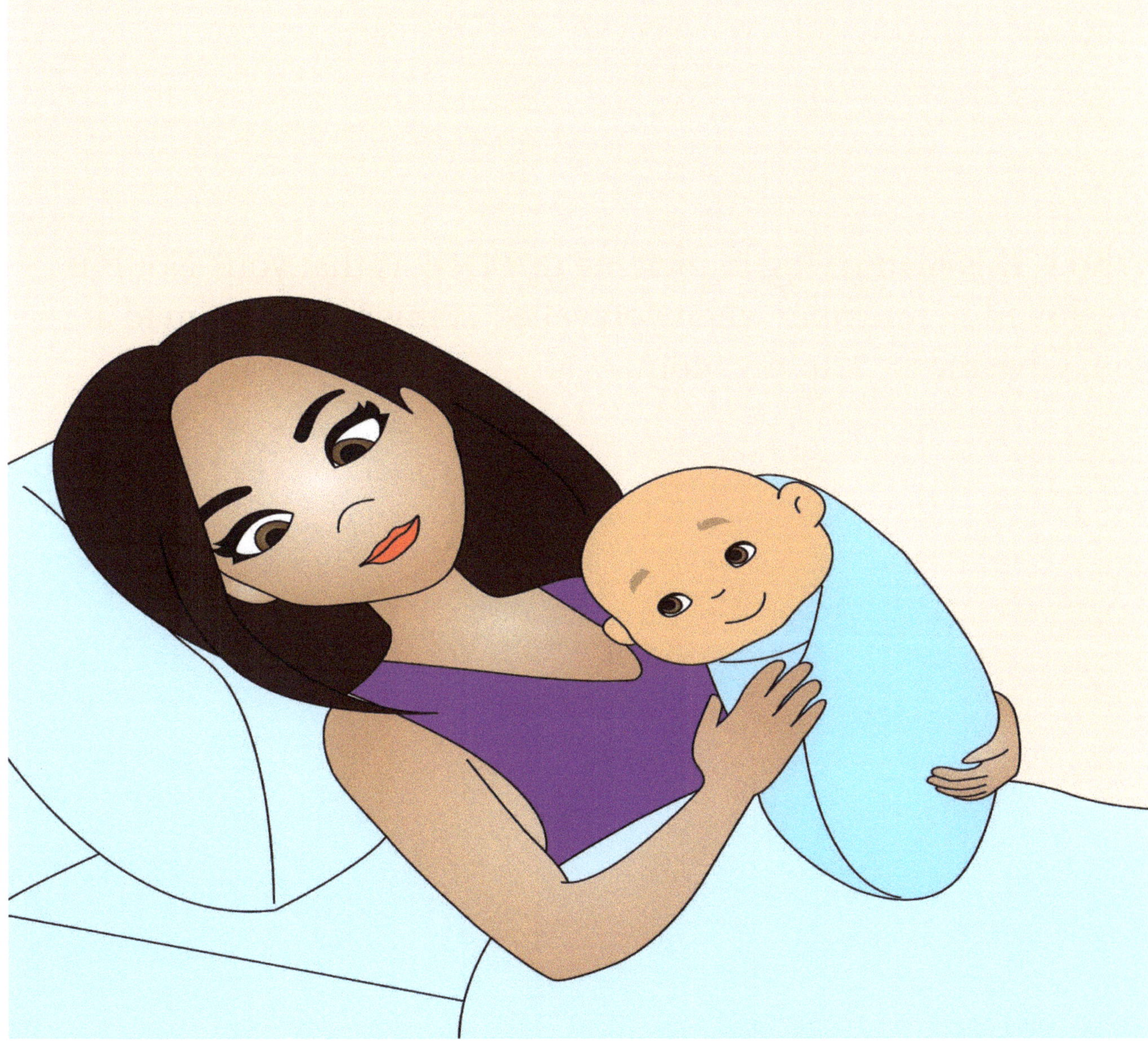

Who is this man trying to pick me up? Dad, is that you? No! Put me down! I remember when you yelled at my mom! I'm mad at you! Give me back to my mom!

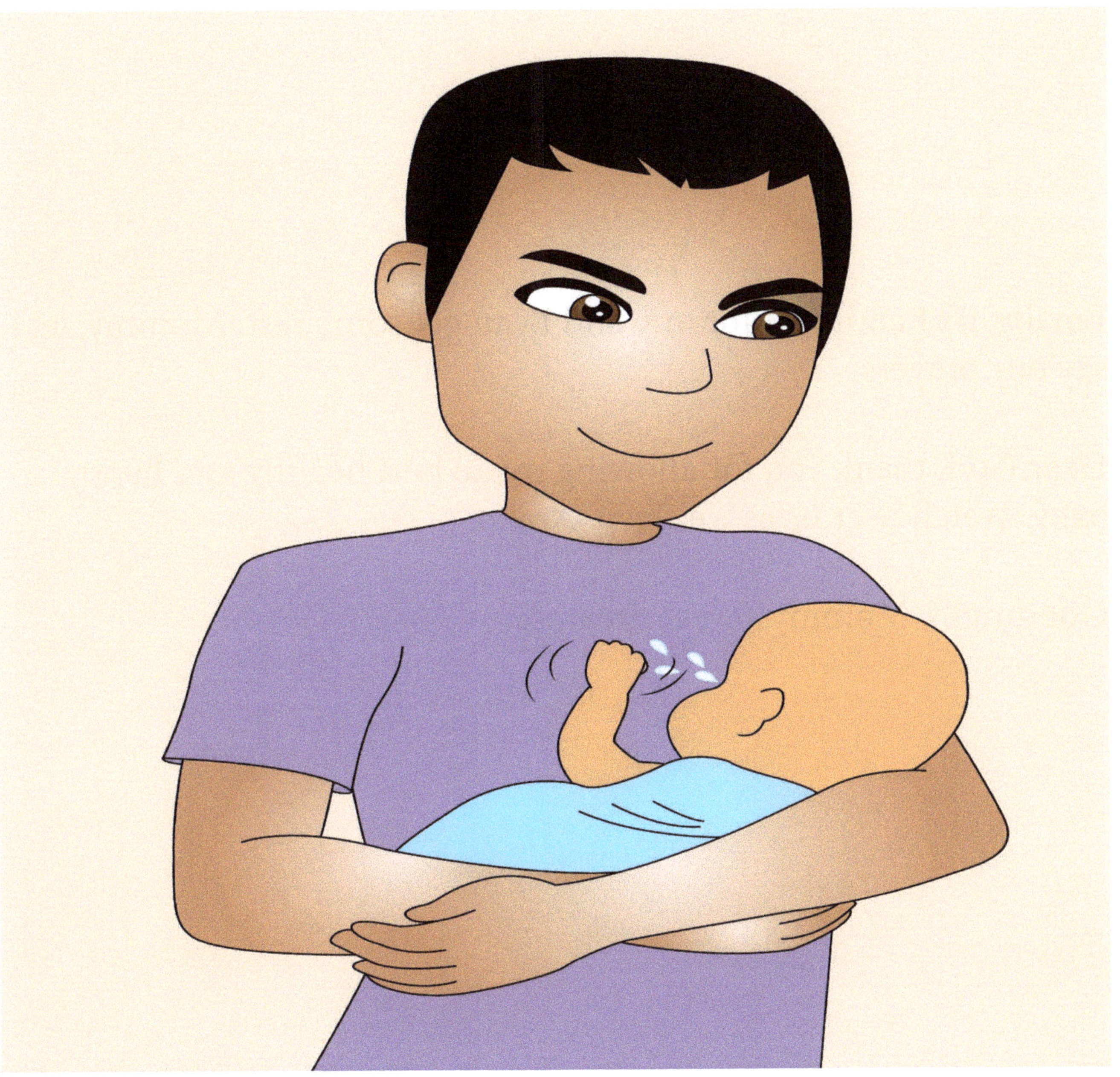

Finally, it's bedtime. Mommy and I can get some rest. Mommy, let's say our prayers.

Dear God, thank you for allowing me to be a healthy and happy baby. Watch over us as we sleep. Amen.

Goodnight, Mommy. Sweet dreams.

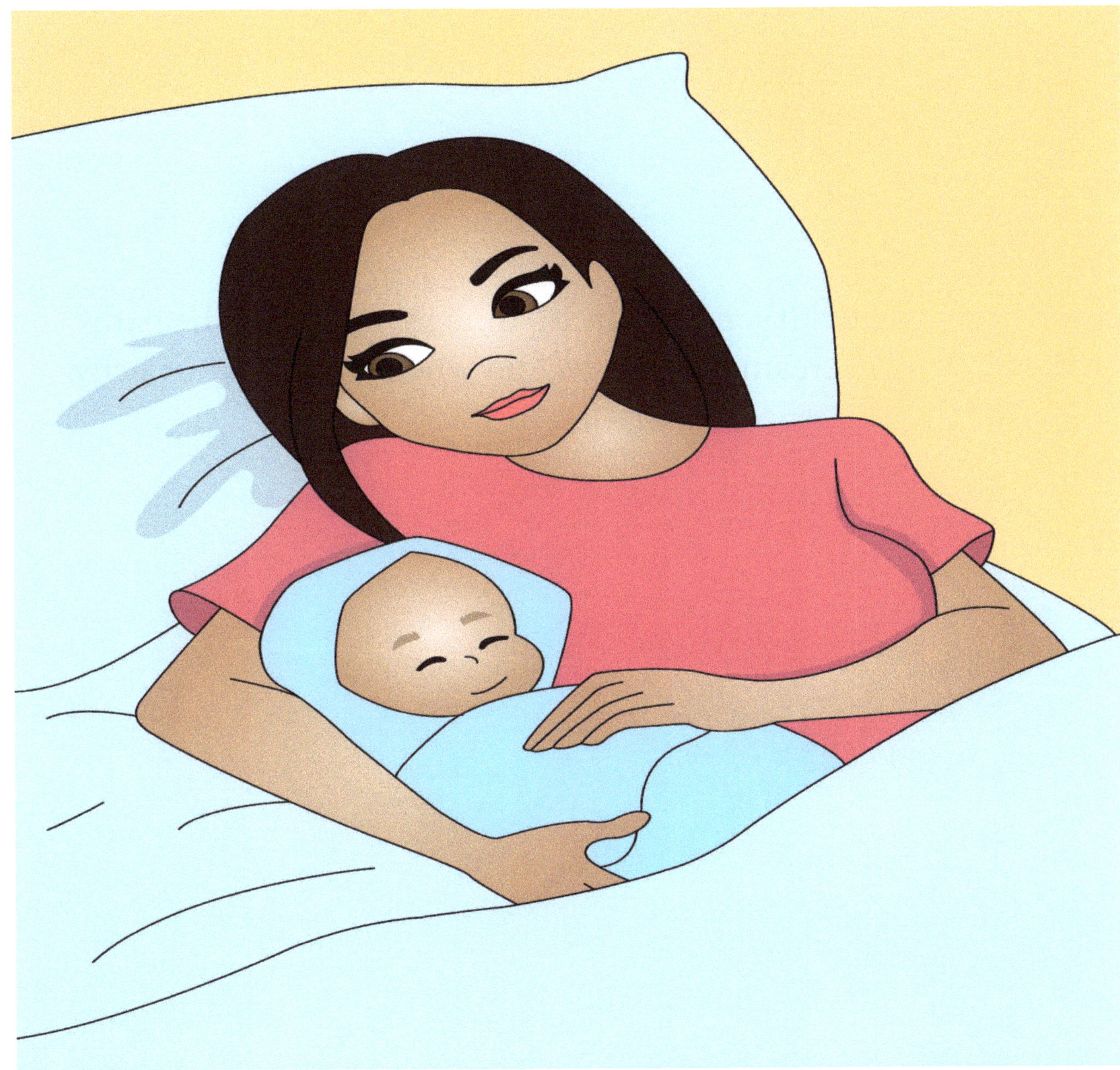

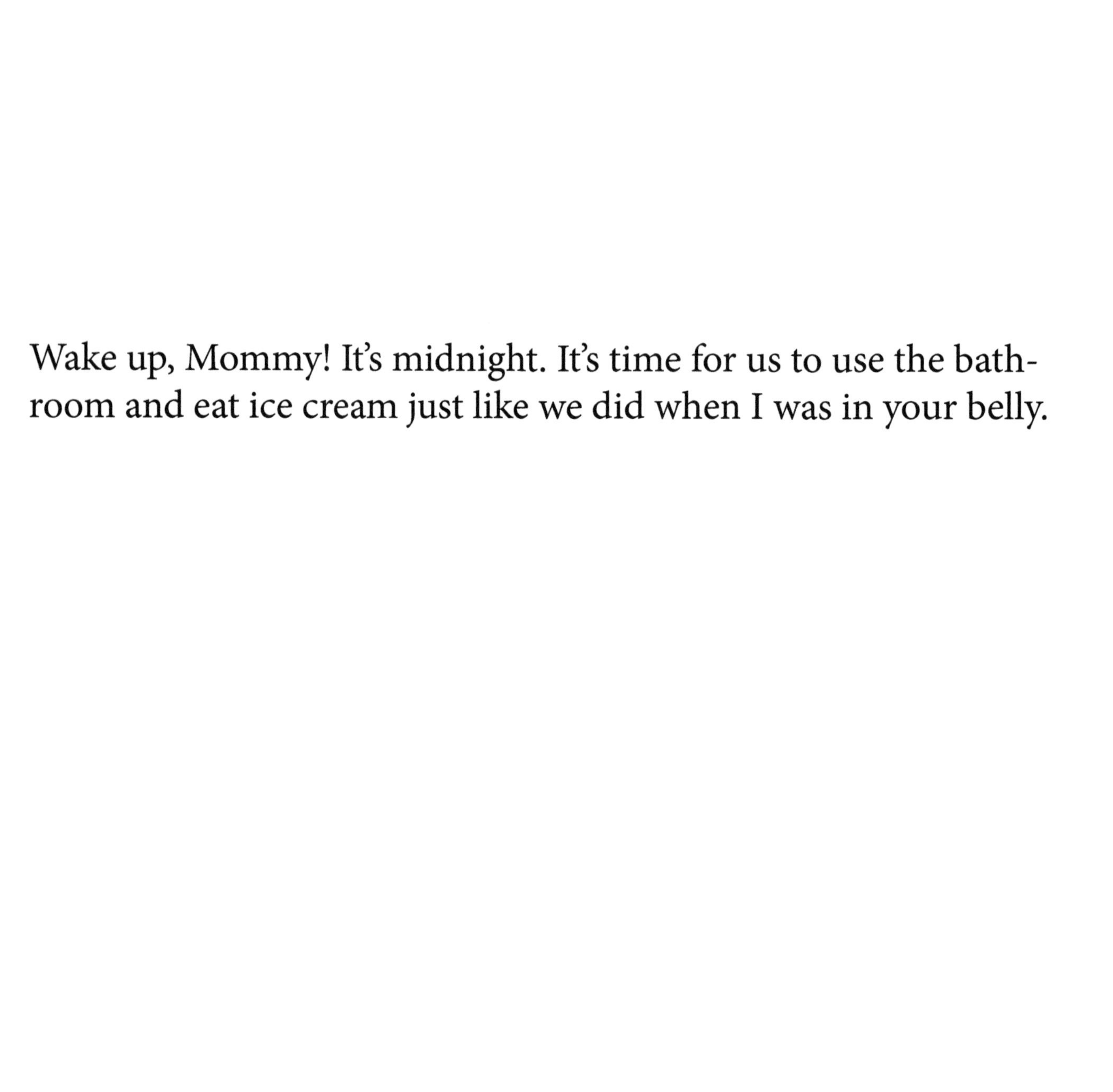

Wake up, Mommy! It's midnight. It's time for us to use the bathroom and eat ice cream just like we did when I was in your belly.

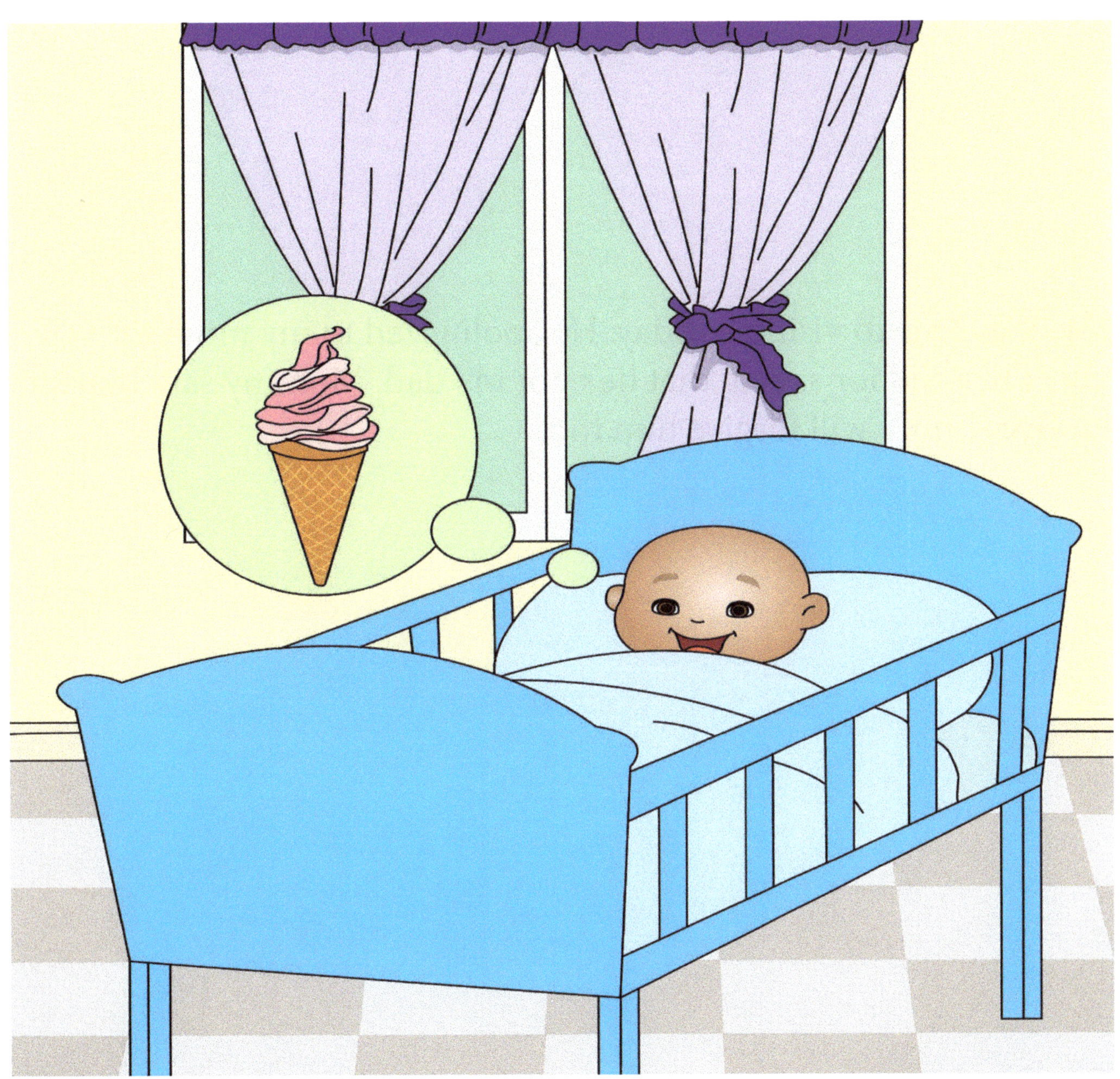

My dad came to visit me today. He apologized to my mom for yelling at her and for saying that he's not my dad. Mommy said that she forgives him. I will forgive him too.

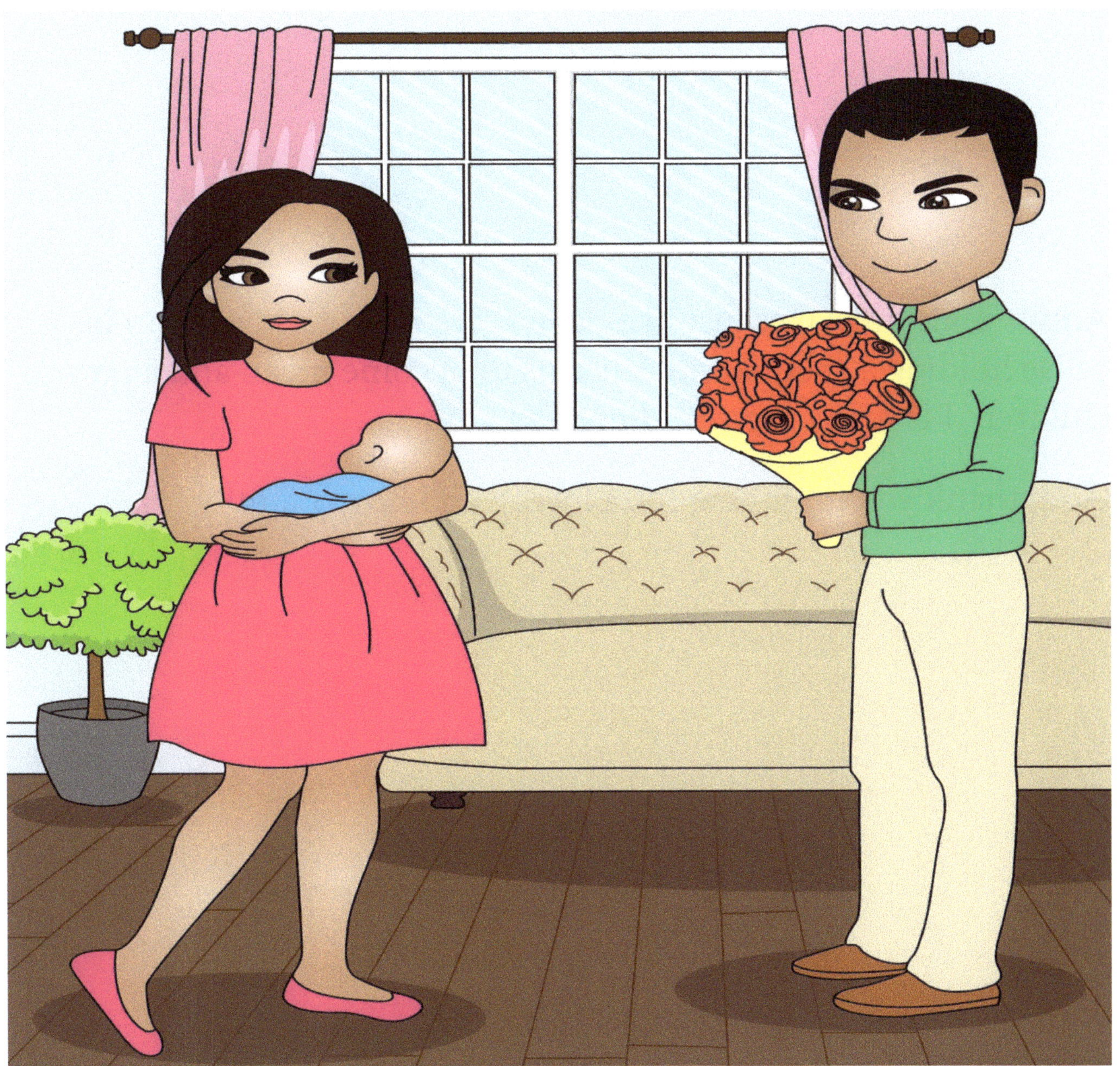

Adults make mistakes just like babies. We must forgive them because holding a grudge will cause us to become mean and angry children. I love my mom and my dad.

God, thank you for giving me a loving and happy family.

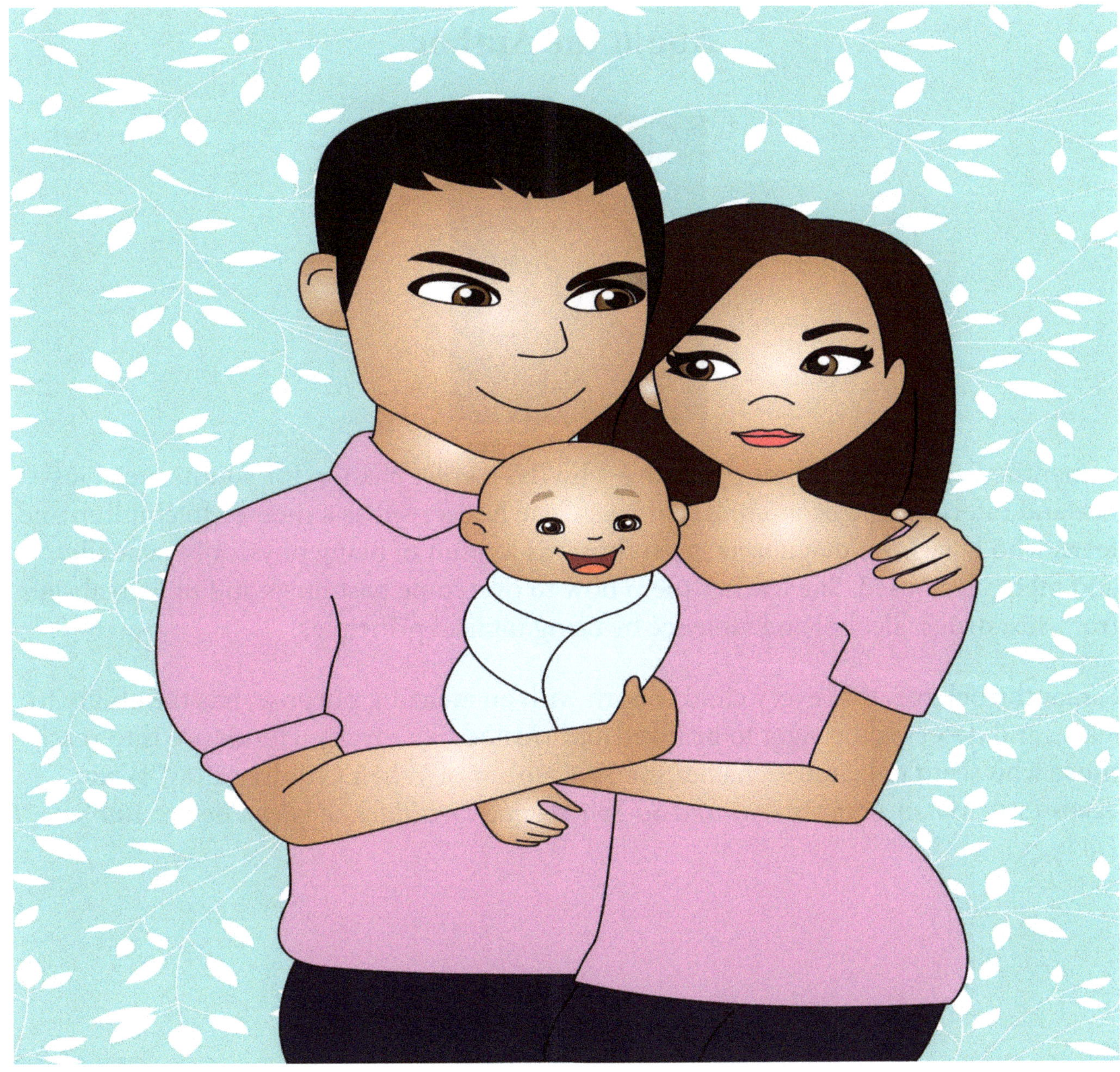

About the Author

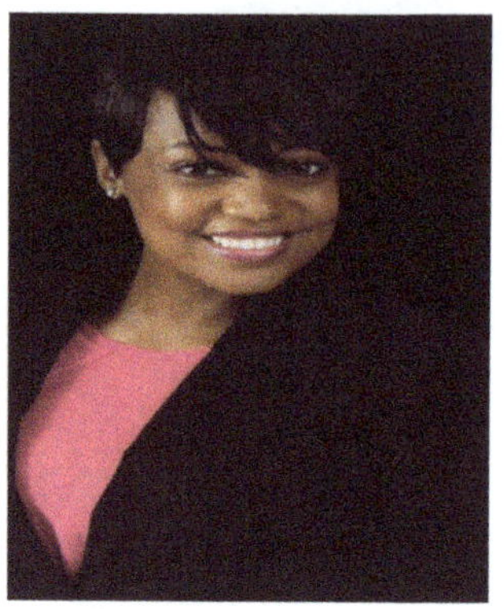

Samantha Pegues is a Mississippi native who has a great passion for youth, social justice and international economics. For years, she has served as a mentor to children and teens who have been diagnosed as psychotic as a result of being physically, sexually and mentally abused. She teaches them how to overcome past hurts and how to abstain from sex, drugs, alcohol and violence by using biblical principles.

Samantha believes that every child is born with an amazing purpose, has the ability to learn, and deserves the right to be loved and treated like royalty. Her desire is to reach those who seem to be unreachable. She's the author of When Children Pray, *When Teens Pray, When Athletes Pray and So You Wanna Get Married? Pray Before You Say, "I Do."*

Prayer Against Postpartum Depression

God, thank you so much for allowing me to deliver such a perfect child. I will not suffer from postpartum depression. I will always be happy when I think about my child. My child brings me great joy and makes me excited to live and love them with all of my heart. Depression is not an option for me because I have too much to be thankful for and to look forward to each day. Amen.

Prayer for My Son

Dear God, thank you for giving me a strong, healthy and handsome son. He will never be depressed or oppressed. My son will not be a criminal; neither will he be a victim of drug abuse and violence. He will grow into a respectful and highly-respected man. My son will be a very influential businessman. Amen.

Prayer for Parent-Child Relationship

God, I am so grateful for my child. I will always respect my child by listening to them and by not gossiping about them to other family members. I will discipline my child when they are wrong. My child will be respectful to me and my household. We will always talk out our differences without using profanity. My child and I will have a positive, unbreakable bond. Amen.

Prayer for My Daughter

Dear God, you have given me a beautiful and loving daughter. She will be humble, polite and very influential. She will be confident in her appearance and speech. Purity, integrity and education will be of importance to her. She will be courageous enough to pursue her dreams and fight for what she believes in. My daughter will be a powerful leader and problem-solver. Amen.

Prayer for Acceptance

Dear God, thank you for giving me such an amazing child. Teach me how to love my child for who they are. I will love my child regardless of their gender. I will be supportive of their career choice. I renounce all rejection that I have passed on to my child knowingly and unknowingly. My child will not be affected by any rejection from the world. My child will be proud of and embrace their God-given race and gender. Amen.

Prayer for My Twins

God, thank you so much for my amazing twins. Teach me how to love and support them equally. My twins will be best friends. They will not compete against each other. They will have equal opportunities and they will both be successful in the career of their choice. They will always love and protect each other. Amen.

Prayer for Favor

Dear God, thank you for favoring me to raise my child. Please give my child incredible favor with you and with people in high places. Teach my child how to show favor and mercy to those who are less fortunate. May your goodness, favor and grace always follow my child and I wherever we go. Amen.

Prayer for Guidance

God, you are the greatest Leader and Mentor. Thank you for choosing me to lead and guide my precious child. Help me to recognize my child's gifts and talents. Show me how to assist my child with becoming who you designed them to be. My child will not stray from the path that you have chosen for them. I will not be a hindrance to my child's destiny. Teach me how to control my feelings and thoughts about who you created my child to be and where you've called them to go. Help me to understand that your will for my child is better than my plan. Amen.

PRAYER FOR A POSITIVE PERSONALITY

Dear God, thank you for giving me a cheerful child with a positive attitude. My child will live a stress-free, happy life that is filled with adventure. My child will not be hateful, racist or prejudice. My child will love and work well with people of all races. Amen.

PRAYER FOR CONFIDENCE

God, you are so strong and courageous. My child is not shy or timid because fear and timidity do not come from you. My child will embrace their unique qualities and not be afraid to stand alone if their peers are heading into the wrong direction. Help my child to have confidence in knowing that there's nothing wrong with them and they are not socially awkward if they choose not to hang around a lot of people.

Amen.

Prayer for Creativity

God, thank you for a prosperous, intelligent and creative child. Thank you for giving my child witty inventions. My child will have the ability to write and produce books, movies, contracts and laws that will make the world a better place. Amen.

Prayer for Mental Stability

God, you created the mind. Thank you for giving my child a sound mind that functions normally. My child will not have to take prescription drugs to stay focused or fight depression. Suicide and murder will never cross my child's mind. Schizophrenia, bipolar disorder, ADHD, dementia, Alzheimer's and any other mental disorders and diseases will never affect my child; even in old age. Amen.

Prayer for Financial Stability

Dear God, thank you for giving me a child who is an economic genius. Bless the works of my child's hands. Teach my child how to acquire houses and land to help those in need. My child will always be the lender and never the borrower. My child will not be oppressed or financially distressed by student loan debt. Wealth and prosperity will follow my child forever. Amen.

Prayer for Forgiveness

Dear God, thank you for my child. Thank you for giving me the privilege and responsibility of such an amazing blessing. Teach my child how to forgive quickly. Help them to forgive me for exposing them to things that I shouldn't have spiritually, physically and mentally; even the things that I am unaware of. My child will not be an angry or revengeful person. My child will be loving, caring and forgiving. Amen.

Prayer for Health

Dear God, I praise you for a healthy child. Help me to live a healthy lifestyle before my child so that they won't have to fight unnecessary battles with their health due to unhealthy eating habits. Give me the strength to take control of my appetite. My child will drink plenty of water and choose fruits and vegetables over sweets and junk food. I command my child's body and organs to function the way you designed them to function.

Amen.

Prayer for Protection

Dear God, you are our Protector. Thank you for watching over us as we sleep. Guard my child's thoughts, dreams and visions at night and during the day. Protect my child from bullying, school shootings, abusive caretakers and all other forms of violence.

Amen.

Prayer for Positive Role Models

Dear God, thank you for surrounding my child and I with positive people who love and support us. My child has extraordinary role models who live upstanding lives and will teach my child how to live a positive and productive life in my absence. Amen.

Prayer for Wisdom

Dear God, the human mind cannot comprehend your wisdom and knowledge. Please forgive me for any words that I have spoken that may cause my child emotional pain. Show me how to carefully choose the words that I speak to my child. Guard my mouth from the use of profanity toward and around my child. Help me to understand that word curses affect my child even though they may not be spoken directly to them. My child will be extremely intelligent and wise. Amen.

Prayer for God's Timing

Dear God, your timing is perfect. My child will not be born prematurely. You created my child for a specific purpose and era. Nothing will stop my child from being born at your appointed time. Destroy every hinderance that tries to cause premature and delayed births. Amen.

Prayer for a Safe Pregnancy

Dear God, thank you for a happy and stress-free pregnancy. Protect my child and I from high blood pressure, gestational diabetes and all other pregnancy-related issues. My pregnancy is free from slips, falls and accidents that could harm my child and me. There will be no complications and no mistakes made by doctors while I'm giving birth. Amen.

Published by: Pegues Enterprises, LLC
ISBN: 9780692085585
www.samanthapegues.org

Prayers for My Unborn Child

Samantha Pegues

www.ingramcontent.com/pod-product-compliance
Ingram Content Group UK Ltd.
Pitfield, Milton Keynes, MK11 3LW, UK
UKHW050136280726
14058UKWH00006B/667